Smart Nutrition Workbook

A Step-by-Step Guide to a Healthier, Happier Life

by the Chef Marshall O'Brien Group

Smart Nutrition Workbook - A Step-by-Step Guide to a Healthier, Happier Life
Chef Marshall O'Brien Group
© 2017 Chef Marshall O'Brien Group

Second edition

The information in this book not intended to be a substitute for professional medical advice, diagnosis, or treatment. Always seek the advice of your physician or other qualified health provider before beginning a new health regimen.

ISBN 978-0-9966293-5-5

Chef Marshall Press
3440 Belt Line Blvd. Suite 103
St. Louis Park, MN 55416

To order, visit www.ChefMarshallOBrien.com.

Printed in the United States of America

Table of Contents

DO SOMETHING TODAY THAT YOUR FUTURE SELF WILL THANK YOU FOR.

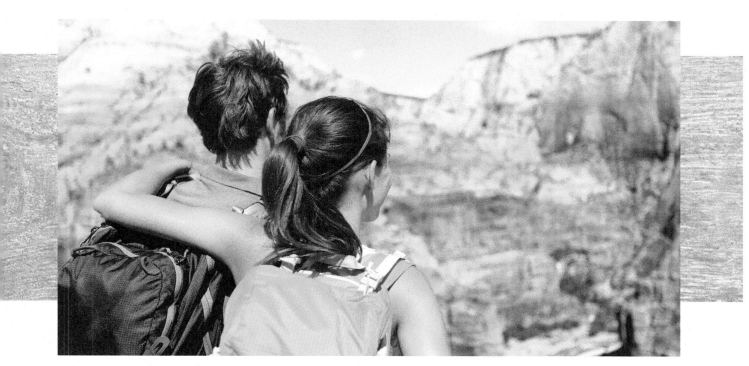

Introduction

We all want to feel better, perform better and live a long, high quality life. Imagine having great energy, sharp mental clarity and little or no stress or body pain. Or not having to worry about chronic illnesses like diabetes, arthritis, heart disease, cancer or Alzheimer's disease. While we can't guarantee all these things, we can show you a pathway that greatly improves the chance of obtaining the positive things you desire and reducing the risk of the things you fear.

We often hear, "I know I am not leading a healthy life, but I just don't know where to start and what to do to change it." We have put together this book to address these concerns.

Only you can make this happen. In 1900, over half the deaths in the United States were caused by infectious diseases like pneumonia, tuberculosis and gastrointestinal infections. By 2010, we had eliminated over 97 percent of these deaths. This was accomplished through actions taken by our society and not by individuals. Cities improved our water quality and sanitation. Scientists developed new medicines. Government regulations mandated inspections that reduced health risks. As individuals, we really didn't have to do anything but enjoy these benefits created by others.

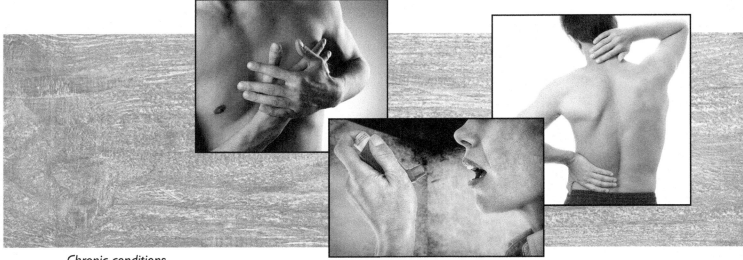

Chronic conditions caused by chronic inflammation

Today, the major health problem reducing our quality of life and killing us is chronic disease, which is the result of chronic inflammation. By the time we are ill, it is often too late because most of these diseases are not reversible. In America today, chronic disease is the cause of two-thirds of all deaths. Half of our population is living with one chronic illness and one quarter has two or more. It is primarily our personal actions that will determine whether we succeed or fail in reducing our risk for these chronic conditions.

If you are not ready to make a commitment to change what you are doing, you should put this book aside and pick it up later when you are ready. Understand that the longer you wait, the more damage chronic inflammation will do and the chronic diseases that develop are usually not reversible.

Whatever your personal goals are for maximizing your overall health, they will fall into one of both of these main categories:

1. **Understand and apply Smart Nutrition to your food choices to help you improve your current quality of life.** Smart Nutrition can give you more energy, better mental clarity, less stress, improved digestion, improved body repair and an improved immune system. All of these things make you perform, feel and look your best. These traits make life safer and more fun.

2. **Reduce chronic inflammation in your body to enhance your long-term quality of life by minimizing or eliminating chronic diseases.**

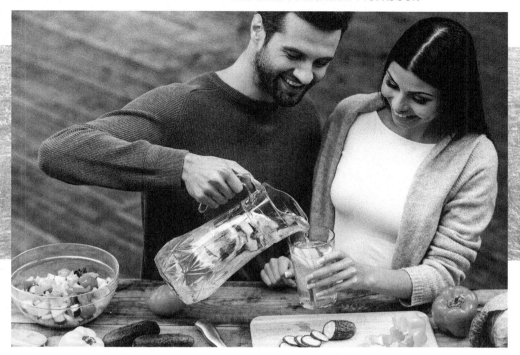

What is Smart Nutrition?

We use the term "Smart Nutrition" to cover four areas that work together to make your life better. They are nutrition, hydration, sleep and physical activity. As you put your action plan together, you will want to include all these elements. In expanding your plan further to help reduce chronic inflammation, you will also focus on some other areas, like behavior changes and environmental concerns.

Understanding Our System

This workbook provides a path that leads to a happier healthier life. The pathway includes this book and the **Chef Marshall Smart Nutrition Meal-Planning website**. This workbook is the road map on what to do. For most changes you want to make, this core road map will not change.

The website performs two functions. First, it has a resource section that provides details on most of the specific goals you want to achieve. We know that best nutritional practices are constantly changing and we update our website to reflect this new knowledge. We are also constantly adding new topics of interest. Second, the website provides recipes and a meal-planning tool so you can easily eat delicious foods that help you toward your goals.

For more details on the website resources, see page 33. Subscribe to the website at **www.ChefMarshallObrien.com**. Use promo code STEP to receive a discount of almost 30%.

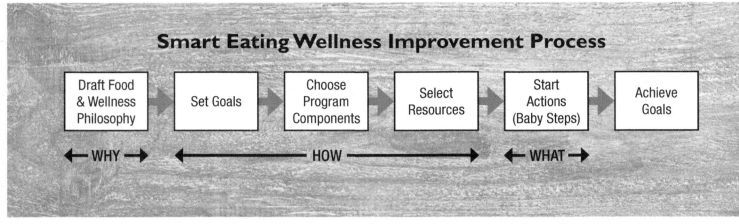

The Why, the How and the What

Why? It all starts with understanding why you might want to make changes in your life and how you will benefit from these changes. Your personal wellness philosophy is the starting point. It is important that your beliefs match the actions you want to achieve. Without first changing your beliefs, you cannot permanently change habits to give you the sustainable program you will need in order to succeed.

How? Once you know why you need to change, you will need a plan. The plan will tell you how to implement your philosophy.

What? The "what" is the specific actions you are going to include in and exclude from your plan. The real work is in creating the correct belief system and putting together your plan.

In looking at your food and wellness philosophy, you will want to include the broad areas of nutrition, hydration, sleep, and physical activity, and for some goals, dental and smoking habits and environmental concerns. Do not think about the changes you are about to make as a "diet". This is the mental trap that leads to failure and disappointment. You need to view your changes as a permanent new lifestyle. If you go back to the old behaviors, you will get the old results.

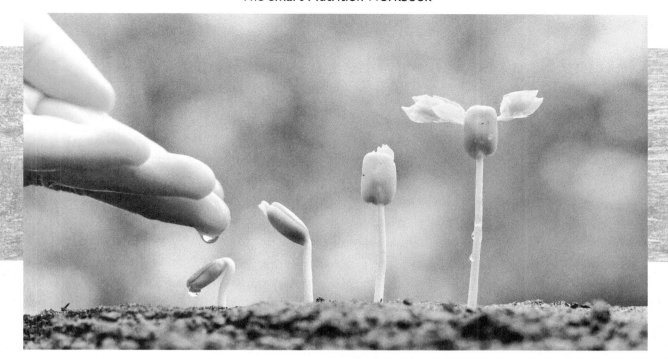

Getting the Most Out of This Workbook

Getting started today is one of the most important things you can do. You triple your chances of success by taking the first step on your new journey now! "Even before I have read the workbook?" YES!!

On the following two pages are twenty-five action steps that will help you, regardless of your ultimate goals. Pick three action steps and start today. Tomorrow, add two more and keep at it until you have implemented them all. As you begin to see success in this early period, you will be more motivated to take the next steps until you have succeeded in achieving the happier, healthier life you are seeking.

Unless you are already clear on what your Food Philosophy is, start by using the sample we have given you on page 12. You can always go back and change it later.

In the next few days, pick 1-3 goals you want to achieve. You will find a list of options on page 9. You should probably start with one at a time, so choose one that will be easy to fulfill. For example, reducing stress may be easier than losing weight. Ultimately, you may have as many as 9-10 goals. The nice thing about this system is that you can always go back and add or change things as your life changes.

Getting Started Now – The First 25 Steps

A. Nutrition—What Not to Eat

_____ Reduce sugar consumption. The World Health Organization recommends limiting added sugars to 24 grams (6 tsp.) a day for women and children and 36 grams (9 tsp.) for men.

_____ Stop drinking fruit juices. Juices are really just flavored sugar water, whereas whole fruit contains healthy fiber.

_____ Stop drinking regular soda, much of which exceeds the daily limit for added sugar in just one 12-ounce can. You can switch to diet soda for the short term, but your long-term goal should be to drink water (sparkling or still).

_____ Stop drinking coffee drinks with added flavorings and sugar. If you want coffee, it should be black coffee, since most lattés and other coffee drinks contain 50-120 grams of sugar. Consider switching to green tea, which has a calming amino acid in it.

_____ Stop eating fast foods, fried food and convenience foods. They are laden with sodium, unhealthy fats and chemicals.

_____ Eliminate or cut way back on donuts, cookies and pastries. The fast carbohydrates and bad fats in these will harm your metabolism and energy level.

_____ Stop eating processed flour products. Minimize foods like white bread and pasta. Switch to products with whole grains, which contain fiber to slow absorption of their carbohydrates. If the first ingredient on the nutrition label doesn't say whole grain, don't eat it.

B. Sleep

_____ Change your schedule so you get seven hours of sleep a night, at a minimum. You may need eight or nine, but start here. If you can say you woke up easily in the morning and were not tired all day, you are getting enough sleep.

_____ Stop watching TV and your computer screen one hour before bed, because the blue light they emit wakes you up. Using an e-reader for books is fine, since the screen does not refresh in the background so it doesn't emit the same blue light.

_____ Avoid coffee, black tea or cola drinks after noon due to the lingering effects of caffeine.

_____ Minimize consumption of liquids before bedtime so you don't need to get up during the night.

C. Hydration

_____ Drink half of your weight in ounces of water each day. For example, a 140-pound woman should drink 70 ounces, or just over 8 glasses throughout the day. This is a general guideline. If you are very active, you may need more fluids.

_____ Minimize coffee, cola and other drinks with caffeine in them, which dehydrate you.

_____ Spread your water consumption throughout the day for the most benefit. You can't hydrate at the last minute. It takes 8-12 hours to partially hydrate and 18-24 hours to totally hydrate.

_____ Check your urine. It should be clear or very light yellow if you are properly hydrated.

*We ultimately hope that you will adopt all of these new behaviors.
You can choose the order you think will make you most successful.*

D. Physical Activity

_____ Don't sit for longer than 30 minutes without getting up and moving.

_____ Use lunch and breaks to take a walk, even if you have to eat while walking.

_____ If your work location allows, stand at meetings and use a standing desk.

_____ Park farther away from the door at work and when you're shopping.

_____ Find a buddy to do your daily activities with. It will ensure that you do it.

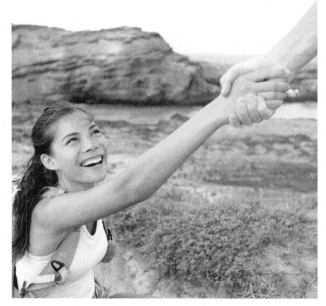

E. General Items

_____ Read this book and put together your Food and Wellness Philosophy and Action Plan.

_____ Find a partner to join you on this journey. It can be a friend, a coworker, your spouse or another family member. Having a partner greatly increases your chances of success.

_____ Learn how to read a nutrition label. There is a lesson on pages 34-35 of this book.

_____ Join the Chef Marshall Smart Nutrition Meal-Planning website. It will be a valuable resource to you throughout the program.

_____ Start a daily journal to track your habits so you know what needs to change. Your journal should include at least the following items, and more if there are other areas where you want to make changes:

- What you eat for each daily meal and snack
- Amount of fast food/convenience food you eat each day
- Number of alcoholic drinks you consume each day
- Amount of exercise you get each day
- Amount of sleep you get each night
- Amount of body pain you experience throughout the day (1-10 scale)
- Your level of stress during the day (1-10 scale)
- What you do for relaxation each day

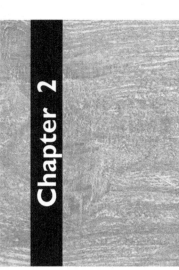

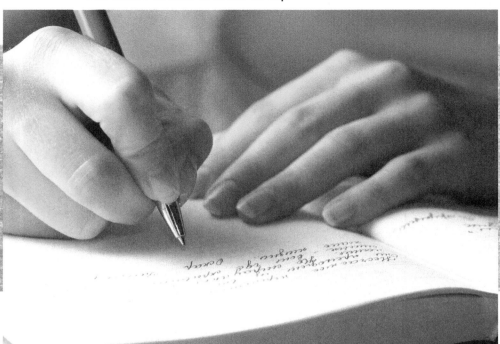

Your Food and Wellness Philosophy and Plan

Your Food and Wellness Philosophy and Plan is a high-level contract with yourself. It is your promise to change. It is not a diet, but a permanent lifestyle change. It contains four elements,

1. your food and wellness philosophy statement,
2. your goals,
3. the components of your plan and
4. the resources you will use.

You need to map this out, because if you don't know where you are going, how will you know when you get there? Your food and wellness philosophy will only become real when you write it down and sign it. The sections of the Food and Wellness Philosophy and Plan are:

A. Philosophy Statement

Unless you know what you want your Food and Wellness Philosophy to be, you should start with the example on pages 12. You can always go back and change it later. Your Philosophy Statement will only become real when you write it down and sign it.

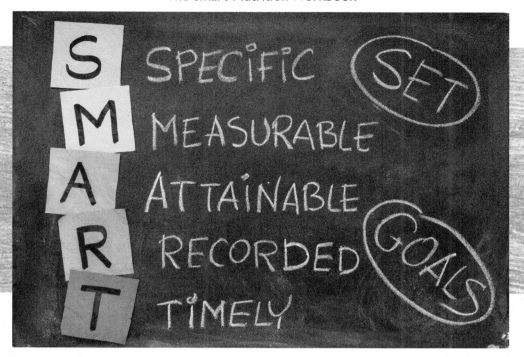

B. Short- and Long-Term Goals

Take some time to carefully think about what you want to achieve—you will probably have multiple goals. Here are some areas to consider:

- Is there too much stress, anxiety or depression in your life?
- Are you always tired and lacking in energy?
- Do you lack mental clarity and feel "foggy" most days?
- Do you live with body pain?
- Are you starting to experience chronic diseases and want to prevent further damage?
- Are you concerned about your children's and family's health?
- Do you need to lose some weight?

Choose the goals that are most important to you. You can always go back later and add new goals.

C. High-Level Plan Components

What will it take to accomplish your plan? List the tasks that need to happen in order for the plan to work.

- Building your plan should always start by educating yourself on what is possible. Only then can you put together a step-by-step plan.
- The next important thing is to assess your current status. If you are trying to lose weight, note your weight, clothing size and measurements. One of your goals should list your desired weight/clothing size or body measurement.

A deadline may be part of your goal, but it doesn't have to be. If you have a class reunion or a wedding to attend, a time component is necessary, but if not, proceed at a manageable pace. Again, this is a lifestyle change, so the plan really should not have a long-term end date, but may have intermediate goal dates.

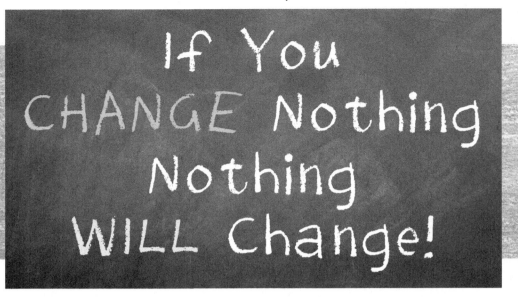

If You CHANGE Nothing Nothing WILL Change!

D. Resources

These are the tools you will use to achieve your goals. The Resources list on page 33 covers this in more detail.

E. Detailed Action Steps

These are the detailed tasks needed for you to execute your plan. They include a start date and a column for end date/ongoing task, because many of these items will involve permanent lifestyle changes. See sample on page 13.

Start Date	Due Date or Ongoing Task	Task Description

Baseline Assessment Form

Date _____

This assessment is intended to help you identify areas of your life where you would like to make changes. You should work with your healthcare provider for medical advice on how these changes may affect your health.

Rate the following items on a scale of 0-10:
   0=nonexistent/seldom   10=very high/very often

1. Your level of stress and anxiety throughout the day   _____

2. Your energy level throughout the day   _____

3. Your mental clarity during the day   _____

4. Your level of body pain during the day   _____

5. Your level of digestive problems   _____

6. How often are you sick?   _____

7. How often do you have headaches?   _____

8. How often do you lack self-confidence?   _____

9. How often do you wake up tired?   _____

10. How many hours do you sleep each night?   _____

11. Would you like to lose weight? (answer yes or no)   _____

12. Would you like to gain weight? (answer yes or no)   _____

13. What is your current weight?   _____

14. What is your goal weight?   _____

EXAMPLE - My Food and Wellness Philosophy and Plan

Philosophy:
I believe that smart nutrition helps my body and mind operate at their full potential and allows me to perform, feel and look my best. Nourishing is different from eating, which just allows me to survive. I am committed to eating foods with the nutrients that will truly nourish me and minimizing foods that work against me.

Long-Term Goals:
1. Apply this nourishment philosophy to all areas of my life.
2. Help my family and friends understand the difference a smart nutrition plan can make in their lives, too.

Short-Term Goals:
1. Reduce my stress level.
2. Reduce my body pain.

High-Level Plan Components:
1. I will find a partner to share this journey.
2. I will talk with my family about my goals and ask for their help.
3. I will learn which foods reduce stress and body pain.
4. I will learn which foods increase stress and body pain.
5. I will learn how sleep will help me achieve my goals.
6. I will learn how hydration makes my body healthier.
7. I will learn how physical activity helps my body.
8. I will do a baseline assessment of my current status so I can measure changes.
9. I will learn to cook or buy the foods that are a part of my plan.

Resources:
1. This book has given me a basic knowledge of the smart decisions I should make about changing my food choices, staying hydrated and getting enough sleep and physical activity.
2. I have decided to join the Chef Marshall Smart Nutrition Meal-Planning website because I can find more detailed information in one place and, if I have questions, can use the Chef Marshall Group as a resource. I also learned that all the recipes on the website are coded, so that I can easily see which recipes I should use to reduce stress and inflammation.
3. My friend, Sue, and I are doing this together.
4. I will keep a food diary so I am aware of what I eat and in what situations I eat things that are not good food choices.

EXAMPLE - My Food and Wellness Philosophy and Plan

Detailed Action Steps

Start Date	Due Date or Ongoing Task	Task Description
10/1	ongoing	Join the Chef Marshall Smart Nutrition website so I have access to articles and recipes specific to my goals
10/1	10/3	On our Chef Marshall Smart Nutrition website, I have found two articles on foods to reduce stress and foods to reduce inflammation (body pain) that I will print for easy reference and use to make decisions.
10/1	ongoing	Start getting 7-8 hours of sleep each night.
10/2	ongoing	Start to properly hydrate. I weigh 140 pounds, so I should drink 70 ounces daily.
10/3	ongoing	Start reading nutrition labels and avoid eating anything that has more than 10 grams of sugar per serving.
10/4	ongoing	Minimize, then stop eating fried food and fast food. If I eat it one day, I will start avoiding it again the next day.
10/5	ongoing	Start eating good fats (from plants), minimize saturated fats (from animals) and stop eating trans fats (man-made) entirely.
10/6	ongoing	Research the recipes on the Chef Marshall Smart Nutrition website to find those with ingredients that are good for stress and body pain reduction.

Jane R. Doe
_____
Signature

10/1
_____
Date

My Food and Wellness Philosophy and Plan

My Food and Wellness Philosophy

_____
_____
_____
_____
_____
_____

Long-Term Goals

_____
_____
_____
_____

Short-Term Goals

_____
_____   _____
_____
_____

Resources

_____
_____   _____
_____
_____
_____

High-Level Plan Components

1. _____
_____
_____
_____

2. _____
_____
_____
_____

3. _____
_____
_____
_____

4. _____
_____
_____
_____

5. _____
_____
_____
_____

My Food and Wellness Philosophy and Plan

Detailed Action Steps

Start Date	Due Date or Ongoing Task	Task Description

_____

Signature

_____

Date

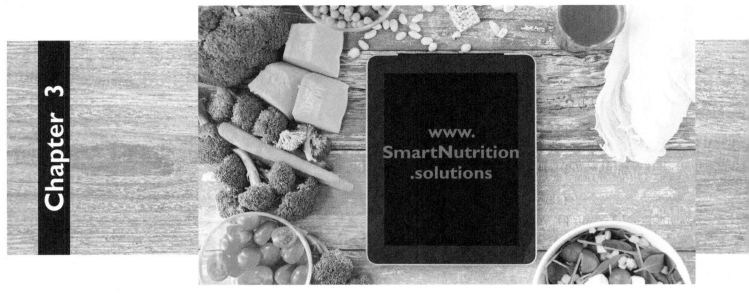

www.
SmartNutrition
.solutions

Key Information for Your Plan

This is important background information you should know before you start to create your plan.

A. Baby steps

Some people are going to want to do everything at once, and if you have a track record of success with this, go ahead and jump in. For most people, if we try to do too much too fast we will get discouraged and quit, so we will be more successful if we make our changes in baby steps. Anything you do today that is better than yesterday moves you in a positive direction. The secret is to take a baby step every day. Remember that you are human so you will have days when you backslide. Don't beat yourself up. You get an infinite number of "do-overs." Learn from your mistakes and modify your plan to minimize/eliminate these backslides.

B. Nourishing is different from eating

Most people think about food simply as the calories that they need for energy and to stay alive. In many third-world countries, this is often the case, but for most people in the U.S., we get enough calories (often too many). We have lots of options for what we eat, so we should be eating foods that truly nourish us. Why would you just feed yourself when you can experience the benefits of truly nourishing food?

You should start looking at all the foods you eat and asking yourself what benefits or health risks each food provides. Nourishment is very important for proper growth and development. Sixty percent of all the nourishment a

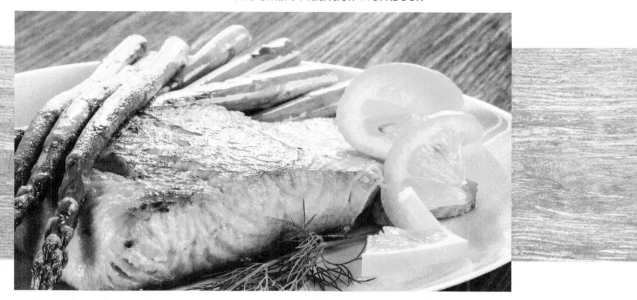

baby receives in his first year goes towards brain development. Children need the right nourishment during their first 18-20 years to allow their bodies and brains to develop to their full potential. Without the right nourishment during these early years, children may be handicapped for the rest of their lives.

And, as adults, what we eat or don't eat affects chronic inflammation and stress levels, and that affects how we feel and perform every day, which ultimately affects our quality of life as we age. Start removing empty calories from your diet and work toward only eating foods that contribute nutrients toward your well-being.

C. Eat breakfast!

Skipping breakfast is a huge mistake. A balanced breakfast is vital after sleeping 7-9 hours without food. It lowers your stress hormones, boosts your metabolism and increases your energy. It also improves focus, memory and productivity. Make sure it includes a serving of protein, slow carbohydrates (whole grains, fruit or vegetables) and a small amount of healthy fat.

D. Portion Control

The first step is eating food that nourishes you. Next, remember that overeating is not good for you, even if the foods are nourishing. It all comes together when you apply portion control—nourish with the right number of calories to meet your needs. You will need a different number of calories if you are trying to lose weight, gain weight or maintain weight.

You will want to eat 5-6 meals/snacks per day so that you are never hungry. These extra meals/snacks make portion control even more important. See page 27 for an easy way to measure proper portion, even on the go.

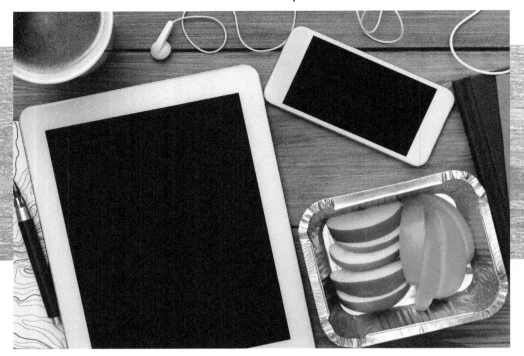

E. Understanding the lifestyle benefits of Smart Nutrition

Foods that give you the right nourishment will also help you reduce stress, inflammation and body pain, improve your digestion and immune system and provide you more energy and mental clarity. Eating a wide variety of foods provides valuable nutrients that help you in so many ways. Learn which foods help you in each of these areas. Information on a variety of health problems, along with recommended foods to eat and recipes, are found on the Chef Marshall Smart Nutrition Meal-Planning website.

F. Foods that help you

Besides eating foods that nourish you, each of your meals/snacks should contain these three components: lean protein, slow carbohydrates and healthy fats. All of these items are discussed in more detail on page 25.

G. Foods that hurt you

Just as there are foods that make your life better, there are foods that put you at risk and cause you problems. The big three offending food categories are added sugar, bad fats and oils, and foods with added chemicals, artificial sweeteners and sodium. In addition, you should minimize foods with empty calories, like the fast carbs found in most processed foods, and excess alcohol and caffeine. Some people who have allergies or sensitivities may also need to minimize dairy or gluten. All of these items are discussed more on pages 21-24.

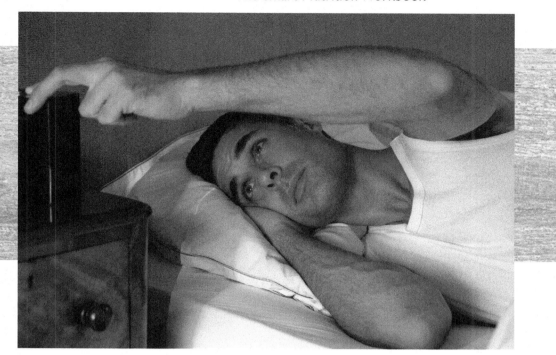

H. Sleep

Most people don't get enough sleep and don't realize how serious this is. Lack of sleep not only makes you tired, which reduces your safety on the job and when driving, but it also leaves excess levels of cortisol, the stress hormone, in your body. This leads to significantly higher stress and inflammation. You can't catch up on your sleep in one night or on a weekend, so develop a plan to start getting 7-9 hours of sleep a night. For many, it will take 4-6 weeks of proper sleep to pay off our sleep debt.

I. Hydration

Being properly hydrated has many benefits. Proper hydration helps circulate nutrients to all of our cells and removes waste products from our bodies. It lubricates the body. It protects our lungs from dust, smoke and exhaust fumes. It is also key for keeping our body core cool so we don't overheat in high temperatures or when exercising heavily.

Most people don't realize that you can't hydrate at the last minute. It takes 8-12 hours to partially hydrate and 18-24 hours to totally hydrate. You should drink half your body weight in ounces spaced throughout each day. While hydrating foods are a great way to get some of the fluids you need during the day, water is the best way to hydrate.

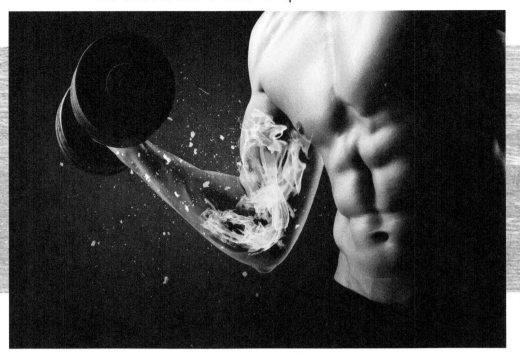

J. Physical activity

Physical activity is different than going to the gym and working out. It involves staying active on a regular basis, all day long. Your goal is to increase your heart rate, which will increase blood flow. Plan to get up and move at least every 30 minutes. This may be as simple as walking around your desk 2-3 times, taking the stairs instead of the elevator, conducting meetings standing up and parking in a more distant parking spot. Physical activity of any type boosts your metabolism.

K. Boost your metabolism

Metabolism includes all the biochemical processes in your body that maintain life. Your base metabolic rate is the amount of energy your body uses at rest. When your metabolism is low, you lack energy and have brain fog. Boosting your metabolism improves your mood, gives you consistent energy and better mental clarity and improves your body's efficiency. If you are trying to lose weight, a higher metabolism will make this happen quicker.

The keys to boosting your metabolism are: Don't get hungry – eat 4-5 small meals and snacks; eat more protein at every meal; keep your blood sugar stable; avoid artificial sweeteners; eat whole grains; include healthy fats; get enough sleep; stay hydrated; build muscle mass and stay active.

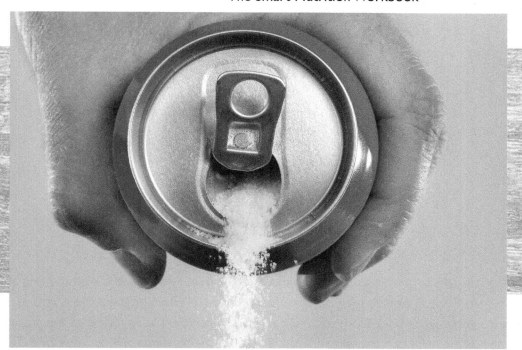

Chapter 4

Potential Action Steps for Your Plan

Your plan will include action items for nutrition, behavior and environment. The items below are some of the main categories you should consider.

A. Items to minimize or eliminate from your lifestyle

1. Reduce added sugar

Sugar is the number one item to eliminate from your diet, due to the inflammation it causes and the empty calories it contains. The World Health Organization recommends that woman and children should consume no more than 24 grams per day of added sugar and men no more than 36 grams per day. As you start to read nutrition labels, you will see that many packaged foods contain more than your daily allotment in a single serving. Besides being bad for you, sugar is very addictive, so cutting back on sugar takes some work.

You need to wean your body off the sugar. Start by not eating any foods that have more than 10 grams of sugar per serving. If a food you eat does not have a nutrition label, you may have to do some research. You will be amazed how much sugar is in specialty coffee drinks, sodas, juices and chocolate milk. When you have achieved the goal of 10 grams per serving, strive to further reduce to 5 grams. This should be your ultimate goal.

Understand that some real foods, such as fruit and milk, are high in natural sugar. Fruit is better for you than juice, because when you eat fruit, you are also getting the fiber from the fruit, which slows down absorption of the sugar and helps level out the blood sugar surge that is so damaging to your body.

White milk, while high in natural sugar, is also rich in nutrients that make it an acceptable drink. We recommend drinking no more than 1-2 glasses of white milk and eating no more than 3 cups of fruit per day. Over 80 percent of all processed foods have significant quantities of added sugar, so read nutrition labels carefully. Learn more about nutrition labels on pages 34-35.

2. Eliminate bad fats and oils

Fats come from plants, animals or are man-made. All man-made and trans fats should be eliminated from your diet. These are also known as hydrogenated and partially hydrogenated fats. They are found in many processed foods, to which they are often added because they extend a product's shelf life or improve its texture. Trans fats raise your bad cholesterol and lower your good cholesterol, increase triglycerides in the blood stream and promote inflammation, thus increasing your chances of developing heart disease.

Be aware that a nutrition label can show that a food product contains 0 grams of trans fats per serving if the amount of trans fats is less than 0.5 grams. Manufacturers will often list an unrealistically small serving size so the trans fats will round down to 0 grams. This is why you must look at the ingredient list on the label to see if the product contains hydrogenated fats.

Fats from animals and animal products such as dairy foods are saturated fats and are acceptable in moderation. Butter is much healthier than margarine, which usually contains trans fats and unhealthy chemicals.

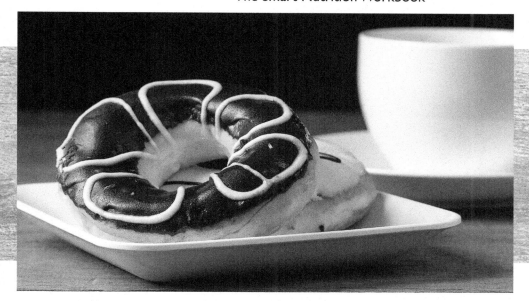

Fats from plants are monounsaturated and polyunsaturated fats, which should make up most of the fats in your diet. These healthy fats can be found in foods such as nuts, seeds, olives, olive oil, coconuts and avocados.

In choosing cooking oils, you need to consider both the type of oil and the way it was processed. Most oils that are used in processed foods, such as soybean and palm oil, are not good for you and should be avoided. The six preferred oils are olive, coconut, canola, safflower, grapeseed and sunflower, provided they are properly processed. Oils are extracted by squeezing (expeller-pressed), heating or using chemicals. Using chemicals or heat extracts more oil but changes the chemical structure of good oils into bad oils. Look for the words expeller- or cold-pressed or organic on the label. If it doesn't say one of these three things, do not use it.

3. Reduce fast carbs

Fast carbs are those foods that contain little or no fiber. When you eat them, they are quickly converted into glucose (sugar), which is quickly absorbed into the blood stream and spikes your blood sugar. These fast carbs are found in almost all processed foods. This includes foods like breads, rice, pasta, baked goods, candies and other packaged foods. Instead, focus on eating slow carbohydrates provided by fruits and vegetables and whole grains, which contain fiber to slow the absorption of their natural sugars into your blood stream.

4. Reduce chemicals, artificial sweeteners and sodium

Our bodies were designed to process real food. In the last 100 years, manufacturers have added a number of chemicals to our food to lengthen the shelf life, improve the color or taste, reduce the sugar or reduce the cost.

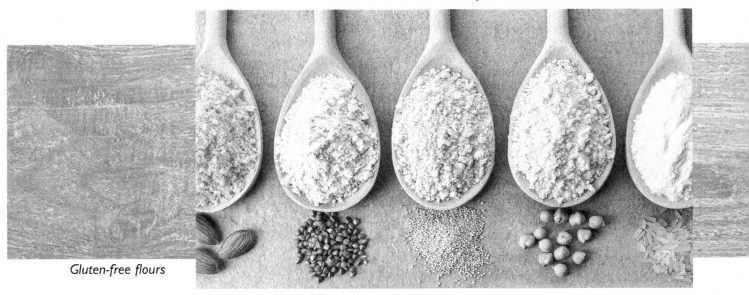

Gluten-free flours

The organs in our bodies don't know how to handle these chemicals, and that makes the body inefficient in processing the real foods that we eat. Strive to minimize or eliminate as many of these foreign substances as possible. Look at the ingredient section of the nutrition label, and avoid foods that have a long list of unpronounceable ingredients. Real food is best!

5. Moderate your use of alcohol and caffeine

Alcohol and caffeine have no nutritional valve and little health value. Alcohol is sugar, a fast carb and full of empty calories. Caffeine can interfere with sleep, cause anxiety and depression and increase the frequency of urination. Both caffeine and alcohol dehydrate you. For these reasons, both should be used in moderation or eliminated. Many people find that, even if they intend to use alcohol long-term, it is necessary to abstain short-term, while they are transitioning to new eating habits in order to meet their nutritional goals. This is especially true if one of the goals is weight loss.

6. Dairy and gluten

For some people, foods containing dairy or gluten are a problem. About one in four people has a gluten allergy or sensitivity. An equal number are bothered by dairy products, and some have problems with both. For these people, gluten and dairy cause chronic inflammation, which leads to chronic illnesses.

If you have an allergy or sensitivity to these items, you should consider removing them from your diet.

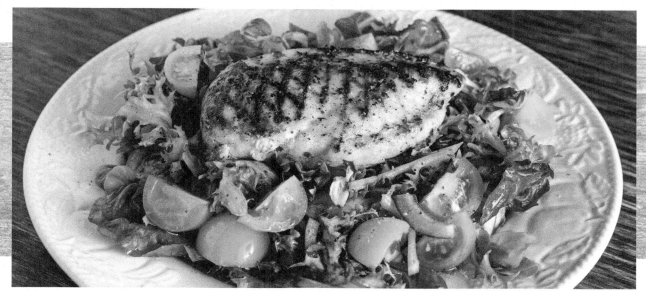

Lean protein

B. Items to add to your lifestyle

Your daily routine should include eating lean protein, nourishing slow carbs and healthy fats at all of your meals and, whenever possible, your snacks. In addition, you want to stay hydrated, get sufficient sleep and be physically active.

1. Lean protein

The goal is to minimize fatty meats and eat as much lean protein as possible. Protein doesn't just come from meat. Dairy and some vegetables also contain protein. Examples of lean protein include turkey, chicken, lean beef and pork, eggs, cheese, yogurt, and legumes (black beans, chickpeas, etc.) Lean meat and dairy products also provide vitamin B_{12}, which is not found in vegetables.

2. Nourishing slow carbohydrates

Slow carbs come from vegetables, fruits and whole grains, which contain fiber to slow down the absorption of sugar. This keeps your blood sugar stable and gives you long-lasting, consistent energy. When buying grain products, check the ingredient list to ensure it's truly made of whole grain. For example, it should say "whole wheat" and whole wheat should be the first ingredient listed. The fiber in these foods not only slows the absorption of sugar, which gives you more consistent energy, but also cleans out your gut, which helps with intestinal health.

3. Healthy fats

Healthy fats come mainly from plants. Examples are olives, olive oil, avocados, coconut oil, nuts and seeds. In moderation, butter and full-fat dairy are also healthy fats.

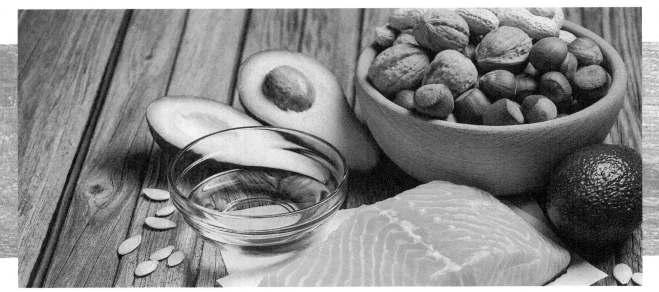

Healthy fats

4. Sufficient sleep

Getting 7-9 hours of quality, deep sleep each night is key. Do you wake up easily in the morning? Do you have energy for the entire day without resorting to caffeine or sugar to boost your energy? If so, you are likely getting enough sleep. During sleep, the body repairs and heals itself, and restful sleep reduces the amount of cortisol, the inflammatory stress hormone, in your body.

5. Good hydration

Proper hydration allows the body to be more efficient in everything it does: digesting food, eliminating waste products, etc. It also helps protect the lungs from dust and exhaust and helps prevent the body from overheating. Drink half your weight in ounces each day and remember you can't hydrate at the last minute—it takes 24 hours to fully hydrate. Water is your best choice.

6. Boost your metabolism

Eat 4-5 small meals so you don't get hungry, make sure there are slow carbs, healthy fats and lean protein in each of your meals so you keep your blood sugar stable, avoid added chemicals and artificial sweeteners that confuse the body, stay hydrated, get enough sleep build muscle mass and stay active.

7. Physical activity

This does not mean you need to work out. This involves just moving as much as possible during the day, at least every 30 minutes. At lunch and at breaks, make sure that you are doing something active. This will really boost your energy. See how much better you feel when you start moving more!

Easy Portion Size Guidelines

Portions shown are for women. Men's portions are about 50% larger.

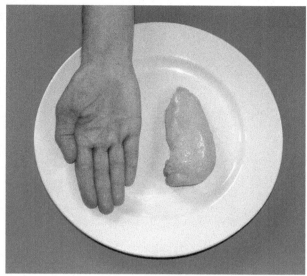

Protein portion should be about the size and thickness of your palm.

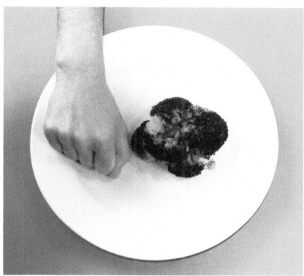

Vegetable portions should be about the size of your fist.

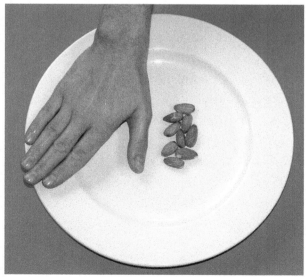

Nut portions should be about the size and length of your thumb.

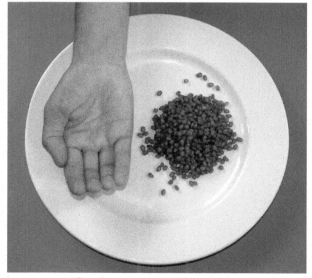

Grain portions should be about the size of your cupped palm.

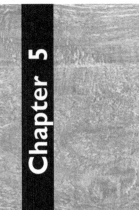

Chapter 5

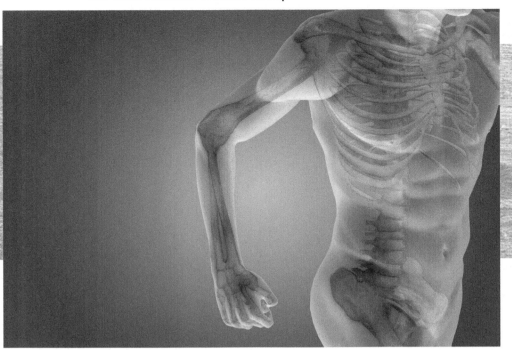

Reducing Chronic Inflammation

Chronic inflammation is becoming the greatest long-term threat to our health, and you probably don't even know about it. Chronic inflammation leads to chronic diseases that currently contribute to over 70% of all deaths in America. We are familiar with acute inflammation, which occurs on the outside of our bodies, because we can see it—think of a sunburn, a mosquito bite or a scrape or bruise.

We also suffer inflammation inside our bodies but, because we can't see it, we usually don't do anything about it. Over time this internal inflammation wears down the body and we develop chronic diseases. The location of the inflammation determines which chronic disease we get. In the blood vessels to the heart – heart disease; brain – Alzheimer's and stroke; cell receptors – diabetes; cellular DNA – cancer; joints – arthritis, intestines – inflammatory bowel disease, and the lungs – shortness of breath.

Once we have these chronic diseases, they are usually not reversible. We live with them for the rest of our lives, thus decreasing our quality of life. Half of Americans have at least one of these chronic diseases and twenty-five percent of us have two or more. While we can't reverse most of these chronic illnesses, we can prevent them from getting worse and, if we start working to prevent them when we are young, they will never occur.

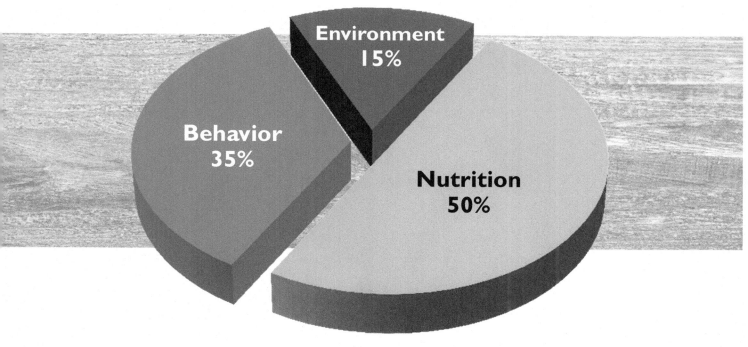

Chronic Inflammation
All three areas need action to achieve real improvement

Three areas affect chronic inflammation—**Nutrition**, **Behavior** and our **Environment**. Below are actions you can take and products to avoid to reduce chronic inflammation related to these areas.

A. Nutrition

Following are the types of foods that should be included in your diet:

- Foods that nourish
- Foods that minimize stress
- Foods that hydrate
- Slow carbohydrates
- Healthy fats
- Healthy oils
- Lean protein
- Herbs and spices

B. Behavior

These behavioral changes will help reduce chronic inflammation:

- Increase sleep
- Reduce level of stress
- Increase physical activity
- Improve metabolism
- Eliminate smoking and exposure to second-hand smoke
- Improve dental health
- Improve intestinal (gut) health
- Reduce weight (obesity)

C. Environmental concerns

Focus on reducing exposure to these chemicals:

- Water contaminants
- Pesticides
- Radon gas
- BPA/packaging chemicals
- Cleaning supplies
- Personal care products

Chapter 6

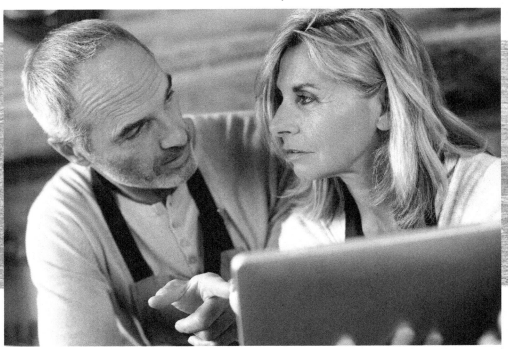

Resources You Can Use

Choosing the right resources is key to your success. You want resources that make the path to your goals quicker and easier. We have tried to put the resources listed below in order of importance.

A. Spouse, family or friend

One of the most powerful resources you should engage is a partner to help you on your journey. If you look at any successful program that strives for change, there is a sponsor, a partner or some other person that keeps you motivated and helps you through times of doubt. We are much less likely to disappoint a friend than ourselves. Find someone who wants to make similar changes or someone who is really interested in helping you achieve your goals. Make them your partner and share your plan and your successes and failures. When you are having doubts or are tempted to make a bad choice, reach out to them for help.

B. Chef Marshall Smart Nutrition Meal-Planning website

Many people have been using our meal-planning website to plan meals, download recipes and develop shopping lists that take most of the work out of making the right meal decisions. They also love the training videos and cooking tips and our videos on what to stock in your knife drawer, gadget drawer and in your spice rack.

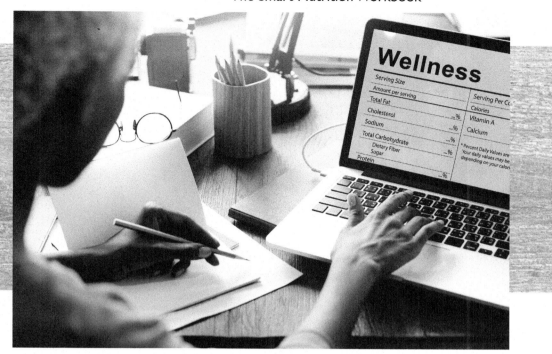

We have added some key features to the meal-planning part of the website to support the Smart Nutrition process. We have coded the recipes to relate them to the problem(s) you are trying to solve: if you want to reduce stress or have better mental clarity, any recipe that helps you do this is tagged with that benefit. We have also supplied nutrition data for each recipe and have provided a mechanism for compiling your daily totals.

Next, we added to the site a resource section with information on the topics/goals in which you may be interested. We have articles on goals like reducing stress and having more consistent energy. We also have articles on getting through the holidays, beating the winter blahs and enjoying summer meals. We provide information on sugar, artificial sweeteners, healthy oils and fats, and on planning topics, such as creating safe zones, portion control and reading nutrition labels. The next series to be added is on specific diseases like high blood pressure and cancer.

We are constantly updating and adding resources to our website. While this workbook documents a process that won't change much over the years, our website is a living document that is constantly evolving.

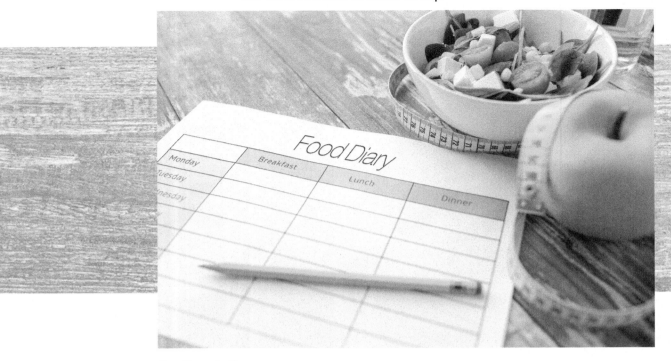

C. Food diary

Eating is often done without thought, and we often multitask when we eat. This is bad for several reasons. When we don't think about what we are eating, it leads to eating the wrong things and eating more than we should. "Mindless eating" is an issue that affects all of us. What you think you eat and what you actually eat are often two very different things. The best way to get an accurate picture of what and how much you eat is to keep a daily food diary where you list everything that you eat in a day.

You don't need to do this for the rest of your life, but start doing it for a month and continue longer if you feel it helps you reach your goals. List everything you eat and drink. Estimate or measure your portion sizes. You may want to estimate calories later, as you review your entries.

A food diary doesn't just list the food you eat. It also helps you recognize choices you make. If you go to Subway, you may find it easy to make good choices but if you go to McDonald's, perhaps you don't. You may always add a chocolate chip cookie to your meal at one place but not at the other. Look for patterns that help you or hurt you and then repeat the good patterns and minimize the bad patterns.

Resources on the
Chef Marshall Smart Nutrition Meal-Planning Website

Subscribe at www.SmartNutrition.solutions or www.ChefMarshallObrien.com

Series of Articles on Functional Foods

Foods that Improve **Digestion**

Foods for Consistent **Energy**

Foods that Promote **Eye Health**

Foods to Minimize **Headaches**

Hydration for Better Health

Foods that Improve Your **Immune System**

Foods that Reduce **Inflammation**

Foods that Improve **Mental Clarity**

Foods for **Muscle Repair**

Foods to Boost **Self-Confidence**

Sleep for Better Health

Foods that Reduce **Stress**

Coming Soon

Artificial Colors and Flavors

Back to School—Getting into the Fall Routine

Fermented Foods

Health Benefits of Spices

Mindful Eating

Nutrients Vegetarians May Be Lacking

Planning Your Summer

Protein

Slow Carbs

SportsDrinks

The Secret Gift You Give Your Child—
    Nourishing Children for Optimal Development

In-Depth Articles on
Essential Wellness Topics

Boost Your Mood (Beating the Winter Blahs)

Boost Your Metabolism

Butter vs. Margarine

Chronic Inflammation (10 pages)

Creating "Safe Zones" in Your Food World

Creating Your Personal Food Plan

Getting Through the Holidays

Healthy Fats

Healthy Oils

Hidden Dangers of Sugar

High Blood Pressure

Love That Produce!

Nourishing vs. Eating

Portion Control

Reading Nutrition Labels

Salt Substitutes - Using Herbs and Spices

Smart Eating on the Go

The Truth About Artificial Sweeteners

What to Buy in the Grocery Store

Many of these articles have companion recipes.

Nutrition Facts

Serving Size 1 cup (110g)
Servings Per Container About 6

Amount Per Serving

Calories 250   Calories from Fat 30

	% Daily Value*
Total Fat 7g	**11%**
Saturated Fat 3g	**16%**
Trans Fat 0g	
Cholesterol 4mg	**2%**
Sodium 300mg	**13%**
Total Carbohydrate 30g	**10%**
Dietary Fiber 3g	**14%**
Sugars 2g	
Protein 5g	

Vitamin A	7%
Vitamin C	15%
Calcium	20%
Iron	32%

* Percent Daily Values are based on a 2,000 calorie diet. Your daily value may be higher or lower depending on your calorie needs.

		Calories:	2,000	2,500
Total Fat	Less than		55g	75g
Saturated Fat	Less than		10g	12g
Cholesterol	Less than		1,500mg	1,700mg
Total Carbohydrate			250mg	300mg
Dietary Fiber			22mg	31mg

D. Nutrition labels

Nutrition labels are one of your best friends when you are trying to achieve your goals. We offer a very detailed article about nutrition labels in the Chef Marshall Smart Nutrition Meal-Planning website, but the key highlights are below.

The label lists the components of the food item and what percentage of your recommended daily allowance they represent (except for sugar). The daily recommendation is based on a 2,000 calorie diet.

If you are on a 1,600 calorie diet, increase the percentage each category provides by 25%.

You will want to obtain nutrition information for your favorite restaurants and fast food shops. Many now offer that information on their websites.

As an overview, there are six things you should always look for on a nutrition label. In addition, the ingredient list is the seventh important item to study.

- **Serving size** – A bag of chips may say it contains 2 servings, but if you always eat the whole bag, learn to double the amounts on the label.

- **Total calories** – If your daily goal is 1,600 or 2,000 calories, what part of your daily goal does this food represent? For example, if you are tracking calories, you don't want to eat more than half your allotment in one meal!

- **Fat** – Pay attention to both saturated and trans fats. Minimize saturated fat and eliminate trans fat. Twenty grams of fat is the daily recommended maximum for a 2,000 calorie diet and 16 grams for a 1,600 calorie diet.

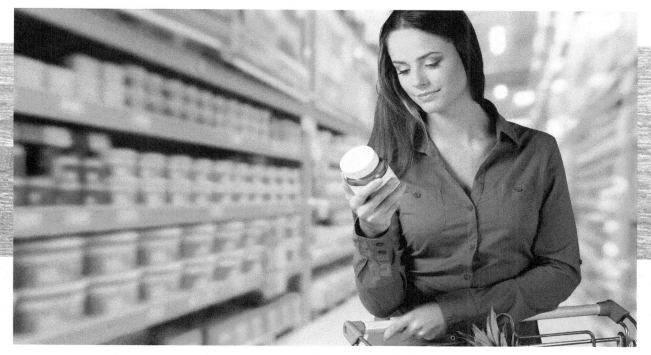

Nutrition labels will almost always indicate zero trans fats because if there is less than 0.5 grams per serving, manufacturers can round down to zero. Manufacturers will often decrease the serving size to get below 0.5 grams so they can round down.

The only sure way to check for trans fats is to check the ingredient list for partially hydrogenated fats or oils. These are trans fats. Anything with trans fat should be avoided, as should fully hydrogenated man-made fats.

- **Sodium** – This is used as an inexpensive preservative and flavoring. Many foods, especially processed foods, have very high levels of sodium. Look at the percent of daily value to determine if you should eat the food. Avoid foods with more than 450 mg/serving and strive for 350 mg.

- **Fiber** – Fiber is good for you because it helps clean out your digestive system and because it slows down the absorption of sugar into your body, which helps keep your blood sugar stable. According to the Institute of Medicine, women need 25 grams of fiber and men need 38 grams daily. If you currently eat far fewer grams of fiber, gradually increase your consumption.

- **Sugar** – Enemy Number One. Try to eliminate foods containing 10 grams or more of sugar per serving and work toward reducing that amount to 5 grams.

- **Ingredients** – This is the list of what is in the food you are eating. The items are listed in order from the highest percentage to the lowest. If you are examining a grain product and the first ingredient does not say whole grain, you should avoid it. Avoid trans fat. Also avoid sweeteners like high-fructose corn syrup.

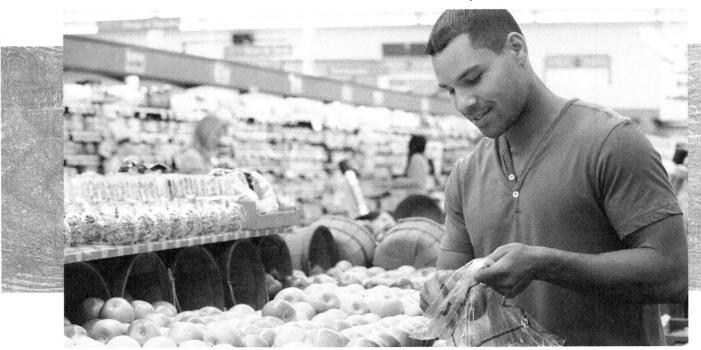

E. Learn how to shop the grocery store

When shopping in a grocery store, you usually want to shop the perimeter, where there are fewer processed foods. You want to purchase "real" food, as much as possible. Try to avoid anything that is packaged in a box, a bag, a can or, a bottle. Frozen vegetables (without sauce) are as good as fresh. Vegetables in a can are often high in sodium and should be rinsed and drained. Learn to read nutrition labels to make buying decisions. The Chef Marshall website has more information on what to buy and what to avoid in a grocery store.

F. Smart eating on the go

We often need to eat food when we are away from home and away from places that we have already researched. These are the times when it is easy to backslide. Develop a list of good restaurant and store options and a list of which foods to avoid that you can use as your guide when you are in these situations. Understand that sometimes there are no good options, so do the best you can.

G. Safe zones

Safe zones are places for which you have a food plan, so you know how to eat. After you re-stock your cupboards at home with choices that reflect Smart Nutrition, your home will be a safe zone.

As you begin this journey, most of your environment is not a safe zone. Over time, you need to change this. You can bring a delicious, healthy side dish to a holiday party or Thanksgiving dinner, thus creating a small safe zone for yourself. You can learn what to eat and what to avoid at restaurants or when you did not bring a meal from home.

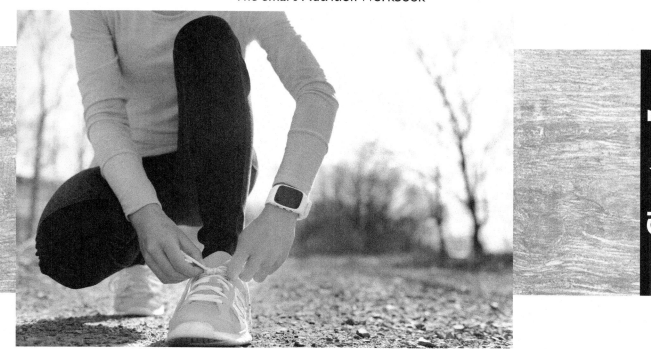

Chapter 7

Implementing Your Plan

Start by committing to a permanent lifestyle change. This is not a diet—you will never go back to many of your old habits. Next, remember that, for most people, this process starts with baby steps rather than by doing everything at once. Start by making a few changes each week. Make the easy changes first, then keep adding changes until you get to your full program.

If at all possible, start by choosing a partner to do this with; their support will make it a lot easier. Next, get support from your family. If you and your family follow very different meal programs, your chances of success are reduced. If your family does not join you, you should still go ahead. When they see your success, they will likely want to join you.

After 3 to 6 months, review your Food and Wellness Philosophy. Update it if your thoughts have changed. If you have completed a goal such as stress reduction, pick another goal and choose your new components and resources. Keep doing this until you have made all the lifestyle changes you want to make. You should start to see real changes in 2-4 weeks after you begin working on a goal.

If you slip back to your old ways after that, you will not like the way you feel. That should motivate you to stick with your new plan. You must keep taking actions that support your goals. You are now that person who reads nutrition labels, looks for the next delicious and healthy recipe, easily resists fast food and processed food and loves the way you feel.

As the years go by, you will enjoy a better quality of life and be happy you adopted Smart Nutrition as a way of life. You will look back and say, "That was one of the best decisions I ever made!"

DO SOMETHING TODAY THAT YOUR FUTURE SELF WILL THANK YOU FOR.

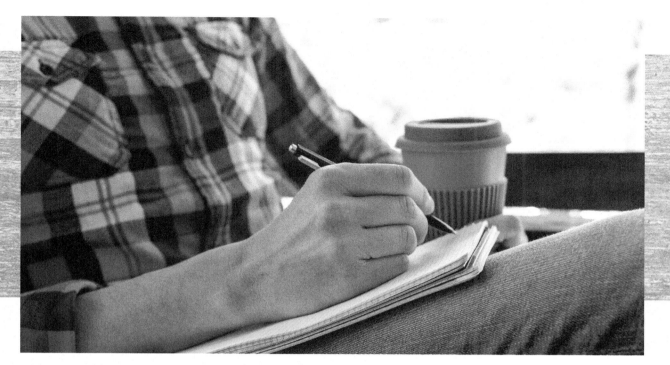

Conclusion

If you go back to your old habits, you will get your old results. To get the results you want, you will need to unlearn those old food habits and learn new ones. You will soon crave the new foods just as you once craved the old ones. Both healthy foods and unhealthy foods can taste great or taste bad. Learn new recipes that make healthy food taste great.

Excess sugar may be your biggest issue since sugar is addictive—studies show it actually stim- ulates the brain more than cocaine. It may take you several months to reduce your excess sugar consumption, but because it is a significant factor in almost every health problem, this is essential.

Getting a friend to participate with you and having your family's support helps ensure success.

Start with a preliminary assessment (pg 11) so you can track your progress. Rate your stress from 1-10. Rate your body pain from 1-10. If you want to lose weight, what is your current weight, what are your measurements and your current pants or dress sizes?

Unless you are an individual who thrives on changing everything at once, remembering to take baby steps to make this process less overwhelming. Set small goals and, when you achieve them, set new goals until you reach your ultimates goals.

We have tried to give you the tools and information you need so you can put together your philosophy and plan to make an easy transition to a happier, healthier life. Implementing these changes is an ongoing journey that will greatly improve your quality of life, now and in the future. Best wishes on your trip!

About the Authors

The Chef Marshall O'Brien Group's mission is to educate and empower people to achieve quality lives through smart nutrition. We strive to teach people that nourishing is different from eating. When we eat nourishing food, we perform better in everything we do.

The group is made up of chefs, dietitians, researchers, writers and videographers. The role of the researchers and dietitians is to understand current best nutrition practices and translate these practices into the right foods that produce the desired results. Since people will only eat the right foods if they taste good, our chefs use the recommended foods to create recipes that taste great. We call this "Putting Delicious in Nutritious."

The Chef Marshall O'Brien Group works with child care providers, schools, the YMCA, fire, police and public works departments, cities and corporations on staff wellness and nutrition strategies that help all people perform better.

In producing this book, we hope we have provided a tool that will help everyone succeed in finding their pathway to a happier, healthier life.

Ver. 4.14.17

CPSIA information can be obtained
at www.ICGtesting.com
Printed in the USA
BVOW05s0438200118
505627BV00003B/3/P